Intermittent Fasting

Heal Your Body, Get Lean Muscle and Live Longer with Intermittent Fasting

Lucy Branson

Lucy Branson

Lucy Branson

Table of Contents

Introduction

I want to thank you and congratulate you for downloading *Intermittent Fasting: Heal Your Body, Get Lean Muscle and Live Longer with Intermittent Fasting*. This book contains proven steps and strategies designed to ensure you get the most out of everything you eat, simply by taking regular breaks from eating regularly. That doesn't mean it is for everyone, however, as it is quite a large decision that should only be undertaken by those who have a clear idea of just what it entails and how it may affect their daily lives.

With that in mind, the following chapters will discuss the benefits of intermittent fasting both in general and as it pertains to several different methods of fasting. There is also a discussion of many of the best ways to maximize the effectiveness of intermittent fasting and the best ways to ensure you stick with for the long term. There is also a frequently asked questions section to ensure all of the misconceptions and half-truths surrounding the topic are fully brought to light. With all the pertinent information, you will then be able to decide, what type of fasting is right for you.

Thanks again for downloading this book, I hope you enjoy it!

Chapter 1: Intermittent Fasting: The Basics

Intermittent fasting has grown in popularity in recent years, thanks in large part to its ability to promote greater rates of nutrient absorption in the meals you do eat. It has also grown in popularity in large part due to the fact that it doesn't require adherents to radically change the types of foods they are eating, when they are eating, or even drastically alter the number of calories they consume in each 24-hour period. In fact, the most common type of intermittent fasting is to simply consume 2 slightly larger than average meals during a day instead of the usual 3.

This makes intermittent fasting an ideal choice for those who find they have difficulty sticking to more stringent diet plans as it only requires changing one habit, the number of meals per day, instead of many habits all at once. Many people find that practicing intermittent fasting leads to real results because it is simple enough to manage doing successfully over a prolonged period while at the same time being effective enough to provide the type of results that can keep motivation levels high enough once the novelty of the new diet begins to flag.

The secret to intermittent fasting's success is the simple fact that your body behaves differently when it is in a fasting, versus a fed, state. When your body is in what is known as a fed state, it is actively digesting and absorbing food. This begins some 5 minutes after you have finished putting food into your body and can last anywhere from 3 to 5 hours depending on the how complicated the food is for your body to digest. While in the fed state, your body is actively producing insulin which in turn makes it harder for it to burn fat properly.

The period after digestion has occurred is when insulin levels start dropping back towards normal which can take anywhere from 8 to 12 hours and is the buffer between the fed and fasted state. Once your insulin levels return to normal, the fasted state begins which is the period where your body is then able to process fat most effectively. Unfortunately, this means that many people never even reach to point where they can burn fat most effectively, as they are rarely 8, much less 12, hours from some type of caloric consumption. There is hope, however, as to start seeing real results, all you need to do is break the 3 meal a day habit.

Fasting intermittently benefits
Building muscle and losing weight are only two of the many benefits that fasting intermittently can lead to. It can also help you to find extra time in a busy schedule as you will find you suddenly don't have to worry about finding time for breakfast every single day. What's more, you will be surprised how much extra money not having to worry about breakfast actually saves you in the long run, even when you factor in the extra amount you are eating for the remaining meals as well. While giving up on breakfast might sound difficult, once new habits begin to form, it will seem like the most natural thing in the world.

Aside from the ancillary benefits, intermittent fasting will also literally help you live longer as being in a prolonged fasting state causes your body to divert extra energy to improving core biological functions as this state sends out emergency signals similar to those that are sent out when your body is starving. A fasting state is quite different from starving, however, and by simply skipping breakfast you soon won't feel that much hungrier come lunchtime once your body has adapted.

Additional medical benefits include a decrease in the odds of contracting cardiovascular disease and cancer as well as a decrease risk of stroke. It is even known to lessen the aftereffects of chemotherapy. In fact, decreasing your daily calorie count by just 15 percent is known to improve your glucose tolerance and lowers blood pressure, improves oxidative resistance, kidney function and reproductive effectiveness.

While the reasons behind these benefits aren't entirely clear, it is likely do in part to the fact that intermittent fasting is known to decrease stress while at the same time making your body more resistant to many of the common effects of stress. This is especially true when it comes to organ and digestive tract health. It also improves how your mitochondria work which makes them utilize energy more efficiently and leave you open to less oxidation based damage.

Studies also show that alternate-day fasting and intermittent fasting are both great ways for those who are likely to contract type 2 diabetes to minimize their glucose levels in as little as six months. Of course, these results were mitigated if those who were fasting used their fast as an excuse to go overboard during the periods they were not fasting. If you want to see results, you have to treat fasting as a regular part of your routine, not an excuse to go crazy once the fast has concluded.

To determine why this occurs, studies were done on yeast cells which indicate that the acritical scarcity created by intermittent fasting slows certain metabolic functions which make cells divide slower which means that it actually makes every single cell in your body live longer than would otherwise be possible. Even with all this positive data, however, what for many people tops the list as the best benefit of intermittent fasting is just how easy it is to get into the habit of doing.

In fact, even in those who are considered extremely overweight, intermittent fasting was consistently shown to be the diet plan that was the easiest for people of all health levels to stick with in the long term. Studies show that they were able to stick with the intermittent fasting on average for at least 90 days in rates that were 3 times more consistent than any other diet. What's more, those who did stick with the diet averaged the same amount of weight loss as those on more traditional diets. What's even more heartening is that 6 months after the initial study, those who were intermittent fasting had ultimately lost more weight than those on any other type of diet.

Rules to follow

While intermittent fasting has been known to produce real results in a wide cross section of individuals, it only works for those who are able to follow its generous rules. These include:

1. *Always run a calorie deficit:* While many diets emphasize this idea, it is crucial when it comes to intermittent fasting as if you are not careful you can easily overeat once you break your fast, and as a result mitigate all your potential results in one fell swoop. Keep in mind that you need to work off 3,500 more calories than you eat every week to stick with a healthy 1 pound of weight loss per week. It doesn't matter how that calorie deficit appears, all that matters is that those calories aren't tallied at the end of each week.

2. *Always be in control:* If you are interested in intermittent fasting then the first thing you need to ask yourself if you are going to be able to go with food for a minimum of 12 hours each day as any inbound calories during this period will reset the cycle and minimize the amount of fat you can effectively burn each day. Keeping your appetite in line is crucial to maximizing success as a single missed meal doesn't provide that generous a

window for the next if you hope to maintain a 500 calorie deficit per day.

3. *Stick with it:* To see the best results when it comes to intermittent fasting, you need to get in the habit of following a set schedule on a regular basis. Only once your body gets into the right sorts of habits moving forward will you begin to see the types of reliable results you are looking for. If you switch between fasting schedules, or, even worse, different diet plans then all you will achieve is causing your body to get confused and cut all weight loss until it can figure out what is going on. Consistency is key when it comes to maximizing your weight loss potential.

While intermittent fasting is known to provide many people with numerous benefits, it is important to understand that it is not without potential side effects as well. When switching to an intermittent fasting lifestyle it is common for many people to experience either diarrhea or constipation as their bodies transition to this new way of eating. It is important to not binge after periods of fasting as this can also lead to internal damage. As such, it is important to always discuss any new dietary plan with a nutritionist or a health care professional to ensure you aren't accidentally doing yourself more harm than good.

Chapter 2: The Type of Intermittent Fasting That's Right for You

While the reasons that intermittent fasting works is universal, that doesn't mean there is only one correct way to go about it. In reality there are numerous options with varying degrees of intensity which means there is bound to be at least one that fits your goals and lifestyle. The best bet is to try all of the options outlined below and see which one your body responds to the best after a few week transition period.

16/8 Fast

To follow the 16/8 method of intermittent fasting, all you need to do is wait 16 hours between your last meal and your first, for men, and 14 hours between meals for women. The remaining time (between 8 and 10 hours) should be filled with slightly larger meals that still remain relatively health conscious. During the fasting period it is important to only consume, 0 calorie sodas, water, 0 calorie gum and coffee, but only if it is consumed black.

This type of intermittent fasting is one of the most flexible options available which means it can work well for just about everyone. Many people find that they can comfortably eat 2 filling meals in the 8 or 10 hours they have to consume calories or, even three regular meals in a shortened time frame. The important thing is to find a method that works with you and stick with it long term.

Most people who stick to the 16/8 split stop eating after a filling dinner and then eat a somewhat late lunch before starting the cycle all over again. This doesn't mean you have to stick to this split, however, and indeed, one of the best parts of any intermittent fasting lifestyle is the inherent flexibility. For example, if you exercise first thing in the morning then you may want to break your fast after you are finished to provide your body the fuel it needs to build strong muscles. It is recommended that you factor the period you are asleep into your timetable as doing so is more likely to lead to success.

Whatever time table you choose, it is important that it does what it can to promote your success, as opposed to be something you have to actively struggle against. The goal should be to follow the same eating schedule every day to maximize your results by getting your body into the habit of burning fat during a specific period each day. If you vary when you are fasting too regularly, it can throw your hormones out of whack, which in turn, can make it much more likely that your body will hold on to, as opposed to shedding, those extra pounds.

If you find yourself in a scenario where you won't be able to break your fast normally, do your best to find something to put in your body to maintain the correct cycle. It is also recommended that you do what you can to ensure your protein intake remains constant throughout your fasting schedule as a high protein diet, 60 grams per day for men, 55 for women, will help make it easier for you to stick to your fast when the going gets tough. If you are exercising regularly you will want to maintain a steady amount of carbohydrate consumption to give you the energy you need.

Meanwhile, if you are less prone to exercise you should instead minimize carbohydrates and emphasize healthy fats instead. If you have a lot of weight to lose, aim for around .7 grams of healthy fat per pound of body weight per day for the best results. Regardless, it is important to stay away from simple carbohydrates, processed foods and unhealthy fats while seeking out natural, healthy alternatives whenever possible.

If you are exercising heavily it is important to always break your fast with lots of protein as well as dark, leafy green vegetables or with nuts or seeds. Together these will provide you with all of the energy you need to keep powering through the day ahead. It is important to ensure you have the energy you need to maximize the effectiveness of your workout and prevent your body from breaking down under the strain. It is typically recommended to break your fast with a moderate meal, then exercise in the next 3 to 4 hours and then consume a second, larger meal once you have finished. It is important to ensure that this second meal includes more complex carbohydrates to ensure you keep up your energy. Remember, slow and steady wins the race.

If you don't exercise every day, it is important to go out of your way to adjust your meal plan for those days as well to ensure you don't accidentally overeat. On your off days, you should focus on eating a larger meal to break your fast, roughly 60 percent of your total, with 1 or 2 additional smaller meals rounding out the day. These large meals should be primarily protein based with lots of healthy fats and relatively few complex carbohydrates. This protein is key to providing the body with the amino acids to prevent it from breaking down muscle in the interim.

Eat-Stop-Eat
If you are already relatively health conscious when it comes to what you put into your body, but are still looking for a way to bump your weight loss into high gear, then the eat-stop-eat method of intermittent fasting might be what you are looking for. This type of intermittent fasting requires participants to go without food for a full 24-hour period 1 or 2 days out of the week. During the fasting period you may only consume, 0 calorie sodas, water, 0 calorie gum and coffee, but only if it is consumed black. It is important to always break these days up and to never try

and go 48-hours without eating in a row. Ideally, putting 3 days between each day of fasting is recommended.

Ideally during this period, you would manage to not consume a total of 3,500 calories which means that once you break your fast you are simply able to go about your eating habits as normal, within reason of course. Especially when following more prolonged periods of fasting such as this, it is extremely important to break your fast with something relatively small and simple to prime the pump for the more significant meals to come. Failing to take into account the proper preemptive period can lead to serious gastrointestinal stress.

Likewise, when following an eat-stop-eat cycle it is important to not allow yourself to fall into a habit of binging and fasting as this is too much variance for your body to handle easily. This cycle only works for those who are able to practice controlling themselves and consuming in moderation, not just on fast days but every day. For the best results, resistance-style weight training is also recommended, though only on the days you are not fasting.

If you don't like the idea of being completely passive during your fast days, then a mild yoga session or some light cardio is all that is recommended. While you might not feel it at first, anything more than that will make it much more difficult to see you fast all the way through to the end. During this period, it is common, especially at first, to experience feelings of anxiousness, anger, headaches or fatigue. Understand that these feelings will pass as your body adjusts to your new dietary habits.

Even without exercising, many people find it difficult to go a full 24-hour period without any calories. While the going will be rough at first, it is important to keep in mind the fact that you don't have go the full 24 hours your first time.

Working up to the full day can make the habit much easier to form and, as a result, more difficult to break as well. Remember, every day you successfully go without eating will make the next fast day that much easier.

Diet Like a Warrior
If you like the 16/8 plan but feel like you aren't quite ready for it to end after 16 hours, then the Warrior intermittent fasting plan might be more your speed. In this instance you fast for 20 hours out of the day followed by one large meal and a smaller secondary meal in the remaining 4 hours. Followers of this type of intermittent fasting believe that ancient humans were naturally nocturnal eaters which means that by only eating during the latter part of each day, you make it naturally easier for your body to process all of the nutrients you need from the things you do consume, ultimately leaving you feeling more full while consuming less.

This type of intermittent fasting even allows a bit of a leniency as during the 20 hour fast you are even allowed a single serving of raw, dark leafy green vegetables and even a serving of protein if you absolutely can't help yourself. This type of fasting works thanks to ancient primal coding in the sympathetic nervous systems which activates a flight or fight response every evening when the sun goes down which makes you more naturally alert. As a side effect, it also increases the amount of fat burned during this period as well.

Following this type of intermittent fast it is important to always break your fast with healthy vegetables followed by equal parts protein, complex carbohydrates and fat. This in turn will provide your body with all of the nutrients it needs to improve and repair your muscles, something it won't have been able to do effectively during the fast.

This is one of the more popular types of intermittent fasting thanks in part to the fact that it allows a reasonable amount of snacking which makes it attractive to first time fasters. It is also popular among veterans for the increased amount of energy it typically provides as the body naturally gets in the habit of burning fat for fuel.

It is not for everyone, however, as it is extremely strict which makes it difficult for people with otherwise complicated schedules to follow. The typical timing of the breaking of the fast can also cause it to interfere with many common social arrangements. Finally, the fact that you have to consume your foods in order from vegetables, to protein, to healthy fat, to carbohydrates is something that some people just can't do. The important thing is to try it for yourself and determine your own results.

Forever Fat Loss
This type of intermittent fasting is an amalgamation of several other types of fasting that even allows you to have a cheat day every single week. To counteract this, however, every cheat day is followed by a 36-hour fast and then a split between 16/8 and 20/4 fasts for the rest of the week. This type of fasting requires a specific schedule as you won't want to exercise during your 36 hour fast but you will otherwise want to do everything you can during this period to make sure you keep your mind off your ever increasing hunger.

If you find it hard for you to control yourself, either during your fast or shortly afterward, then this is likely not the right type of fasting for you as it can be difficult to avoid binging after so long without food. You must have complete control over yourself at all times for this type of fasting to be effective as moving in on direction will cause you to overate and not lose weight and moving in the other direction can lead to physical harm due to malnourishment.

For those who can build up to this level of tolerance, however, this type of fasting is known to burn more fat per fasting period than any other type of fasting. It is important to monitor your caloric and nutritional intake carefully, however, as it is easy to get out of line and accidentally cause yourself more harm than good if you are not extremely careful. During the 36-hour period you may have one serving of healthy dark leafy green vegetables as well as 0 calorie sodas, water, 0 calorie gum and coffee, but only if it is consumed black. Coffee or 0 calorie soda is recommended to combat the feelings of hunger you will otherwise most certainly feel.

Alternating Fasting

If you find that you have trouble going 12 hours without eating without feeling practically sick from hunger, then the alternating method of intermittent fasting may be right for you. In this method of intermittent fasting you simply eat regularly one day and then eat 20 percent of your average caloric consumption then next, followed by another normal day and so on. Ideally your will be somewhere around 400 calories on your "fast" days, though if you typically consume more than 2,000 calories per day then always err on the side of more calories as consuming too few calories won't do you any good and can actually cause your body long lasting harm from malnutrition.

Many people find this type of intermittent fasting effective and stick to a variety of filling protein shakes to get them through their low calorie days. This is only recommended to get you started, however, and working back to nutritious whole foods on your low calorie days are recommended to keep your nutrition level where it ultimately needs to be. This is one of the more effective forms of intermittent fasting weight loss and a maximum of 2 lbs. per week have been reported. It is important to understand that that will not last in the long term, however, and eventually 1 pound per week lost is considered healthy.

Irregular fasting

If you are curious how your body will react but don't want to commit to anything major, then skipping meals for 12 hours at a time now and then may be the best choice for you. While you won't see the same variety of benefits you would if you stuck to a more permanent schedule, you will be able to see how your body reacts to the process in terms of hunger and energy levels which may make it easier to commit fully at some point in the future.

This doesn't mean you won't see some benefits and many of the health benefits will come along intact as well. With so many types of intermittent fasting, practicing occasionally makes it much more likely you will ultimately end up with a plan that sticks, regardless of your unique or uncompromising schedule. After all, you have, literally, nothing to lose but a little unwanted weight.

Chapter 3: Ways to Get the Most Out of Intermittent Fasting

Just because intermittent fasting is undeniably beneficial, doesn't mean that it can't be quite difficult to get the hang of, or to follow through on in the long term. Consider the following suggestions as guideposts on your path to success and remember, it is best to think of intermittent fasting as a journey, not a destination.

Be honest with yourself: Just because intermittent fasting might offer the sorts of health benefits that you are looking for, it doesn't mean that it is automatically the right choice for you. While you might be able to make it through one or two fasts without issue, it is important to ask yourself if your internal and external factors are going to realistically align in such a way as to make intermittently fasting on the regular a viable proposition.

Think about how disciplined you really are, what your relationship with food is like and how healthy you are in general. If you are looking for a way to get started down a healthier path for the first time, perhaps something with a less clearly defined failure state might be in order. Remember, it is a lot easier to be realistic about your chance of success and decide to look elsewhere before you get started in earnest than after struggling with and failing at fasting after a week or more of serious effort.

Be aware of your body's response: While you will want to monitor how your body is reacting to the intermittent fasting process as long as you are regularly withholding calories, this is especially important during the first month while your body is transitioning to a new way of receiving calories. While you may feel faint, lightheaded, shaky, irritable, angry or weak for up to a month while fasting, symptoms that persist indefinitely are a sign that something ultimately isn't right. It is important to be in touch with your body enough to know when it's time to consult a health care professional.

Don't expect constant weight loss: While you will likely see weight loss at first as your body adapts to fewer calories in its system on average; this will likely start and stop throughout your time fasting, especially after the first few weeks of the transition as your body tries to hold on to everything it has until it can figure out what is going on. Once it gets with the program, however, things should proceed as expected.

Every diet is going to have periods of weight loss plateau, that is simply a part of weight loss that cannot be mitigated. As long as you stay consistent weight loss will eventually resume. The worst thing you can do is to try and change things up to get weight loss back on track as that will only make it more difficult for your body to start shedding weight once more.

Drink lots of water: This doesn't mean simply stay hydrated, which is good advice regardless, it means drink at minimum a gallon of water each day. It will help you feel full and also ensure your body continues processing toxins normally, even if it is holding onto all of its fat due to the transition that is occurring. This is a good exercise for most people anyway, as roughly 40 percent of adults are walking around right now in a mild state of dehydration. In fact, if thirst remains untreated for long enough, it actually starts manifesting itself as hunger so staying hydrated will actually keep you feeling more full longer in two ways.

Use caffeine like a tool: Especially when you first begin training your body to expect food less often, drinking black coffee or a 0 calorie soda every 3 or 4 hours can make it easier to get through the early fasts as caffeine is known to actively suppress the appetite. It is important to not go overboard, however, as many artificial sweeteners have been known to cause health problems when consumed in large amounts. In addition, it is important to not begin to rely on caffeine to the point that your body doesn't actually adapt to the fasting schedule. Feel free to use as much caffeine as you need to get through the first few days of fasting, but keep your intake under control from there as you want your body to be building new habits, not simply have its appetite stunted by caffeine.

Plan on keeping busy: While this is a good suggestion in general when it comes to the final few hours of your fast, it is especially important during your transition period. Having nothing to do but sit around for several hours until you can eat again is a surefire way to put your untrained body into a situation it can't help but fail in. Don't let this happen to you, ensure your fast will break after a period of constant mental activity and you will find those last few hours flying by.

Plan with fasting in mind: It is important to take into account when your body and mind are at their peak fuel wise, and schedule accordingly. You should start each day with the most difficult task you have to accomplish as it will only get more difficult to consider tackling as the day goes on. Your body will naturally begin to slow down across the board in an effort to preserve energy once the fasting period really begins, know what you are in for and understand your limits if you want to guarantee success.

Don't make excuses: It is important to not let reasons for not starting an intermittent fast turn into excuses. For example, having a busy schedule or not being able to work in a 12-hour fast are simply reasons that your brain is coming up with to allow you to not try something hard without feeling bad about crying off. The only person who can ensure you are motivated enough to make intermittent fasting work is you, commit to success and follow through on your weight loss goals.

Be realistic: It is important to not expect results right away, remember 3,500 calories not consumed is only equal to 1 pound of fat. If you find yourself getting discouraged by your lack of apparent results, take the time to consider how long it took for you to reach your current weight and cut yourself some slack. It is only reasonable to expect a similar amount of effort and commitment to be required to reach your weight loss goals.

Don't stick with the first plan you try: There are numerous types of intermittent fasting that you can try as well as several different patterns you can try when it comes to on/off patterns and the number, size and frequency of the meals that you do eat. Don't underestimate the importance of any one of these options and mix and match a variety of fasting styles and times to see what your body responds to best. Even if the first option you try seems acceptable, you never know if something even better might be waiting to blow you away.

Don't forget BCAA: Branch chain amino acids are an important supplement to consider if you are planning to fast for 24 to 36 hours on a regular basis. Remember, it is important to never attempt to fast for more than 36 hours at once. BCAA supplements will stimulate additional weight loss while at the same time ensuring that your lean muscle won't be broken down while your body looks for nutrients during your fast.

Take it slow: If you have never gone more than a few hours without eating, then it is a good idea to start out slowly, by going 10 hours without eating and then build up your tolerance from there. It is important to go slow, as if you experience lots of failure early on, it can be more difficult to convince your brain to get into a pro-fasting mindset in the long term. Once you begin to see real weight loss results you will notice that it will become easier to persevere, all you have to do is make it to that point and things will begin to fall into place.

Be discrete: While the scientific evidence to support it is readily available, many people still have a flawed view of intermittent fasting that can be difficult to deal with while your body is already going through the transition period. As such, it is best to keep your new diet to yourself until you have the readily available proof that can crush any negativity that might otherwise come your way. You know what you are up to and what the potential benefits are, let that be enough to get you through the rocky start.

Give yourself a break: When first starting out, it is important to understand that the transition period can be rather difficult, and it will be worse for some people than others. As such, it is a good idea to choose a time to start the transition that is relatively free from stress or otherwise hectic plans. You are likely going to have a hard enough making the transition that anything else on your plate is likely going to take a hit. Forewarned is forearmed, however and planning for the transition will make it easier to manage.

Reward yourself: Especially when you are first starting out, it is important to reward a successful week of fasting with some type of splurge. As long as you don't let it get out of hand, there is no harm in having an extra decadent dessert, remember you only need to cut out 3,500 calories to lose a pound, as long as you make it up elsewhere there is no need to hold yourself to the highest standards right away. Instead, consider how successful you have already been and understand that your brain is likely to link intermittent fasting with a delayed reward which means it will be easier to persevere in the long run.

Eat more protein: If, after the transition period ends you still find yourself hungry long before your fast is scheduled to be broken, then you are likely not eating enough protein in your diet. Aside from red meat, poultry and fish, nuts are a great source of protein as are beans. If you still can't get enough, consider protein powders, shakes or bars in the short term though natural options are a better choice in the long term as they are typically more nutritious as a whole.

Avoid junk food: While intermittent fasting means that you will likely have a little extra caloric room in your diet for junk food if you so choose, trying to eat poorly while intermittent fasting will only lead to failure. While you may technically be able to spare the calories, spending the ones you do have on things that won't stick to your ribs for the long haul is a recipe for disaster. Focus on foods that are high in protein and healthy fats and you will feel more full and energetic for longer periods every time. You only have so much time you can eat each day, make it count.

Understand when you are really hungry: Especially early on in the transition, you will likely find that you are hungry right about the time you previously ate breakfast, lunch and dinner. While there is likely some physical truth to that hunger, odds are it is primarily in your head. The habits that you held before will continue to befuddle you for a time but eventually they will fade and you will find that in reality you weren't nearly as hungry as you previously thought. It is important to distinguish between the two types of hunger as true and serious feelings of the true sort should always be enough to bring an early end to any fast.

Fast appropriately: If you are considering using intermittent fasting as a way to cover up a prolonged desire to not eat a healthy amount of calories in a day, then it is strongly recommended that you reconsider. Before you attempt intermittent fasting it is important to know that you have the willpower, not just to prevent yourself from eating, but also to force yourself to never push your limits to the point that your safety can be called into question. Also practice intermittent fasting safely and in a healthy moderation.

Chapter 4: Intermittent Fasting FAQ

While the previous chapters have done what they can to elucidate the merits and potential dangers of intermittent fasting, there are always going to be a few questions that slip through the cracks. Consider the following frequently asked questions before making your final decision as to whether or not intermittent fasting is the right choice for you, right now.

If I am currently on another diet, can I stop it and start intermittent fasting right away?

Because intermittent fasting is not a diet in the traditional sense, there is no reason that you cannot combine it with your favorite diet of choice as long as they are not inherently incompatible. Don't forget to consider how the other diet handles metabolism, however, as it may not then work with a large gap between meals. Other than that, it is only important that your body has finished adapting to your current diet before you ask it to begin adapting to another one.

How do I make it through the morning without breakfast?

If you find yourself feeling excessively hungry in the early morning hours, the first thing you should keep in mind is that much of this hunger is actually mental, rather than physical. After you have finished the transition you should notice it much less often. With that being said, it is important to start each day by drinking a liter of water; and a cup of black coffee is a good idea as well. If, after all of that, you still feel hungry, consider ending your previous day's meal with extra protein and healthy fats which should stick with you through morning.

How should I structure the meals I do eat?

One of the best parts of most types of intermittent fasting is that there is no right way to break your fast as long as you don't binge or eat too much, too fast. Don't worrying about trying to limit yourself to artificial patterns, simply eat healthy foods that you want to eat and stop once you feel full. If you are really sticking to the types of natural, healthy foods that you should try and consume then it is hard to eat too much of them without feeling full first. Always try and listen to your body first and foremost and make additional decision from there.

Is it safe to exercise while intermittently fasting?

As long as you take into account the amount of calories you have to burn each day, there is no reason that you cannot successfully integrate your current exercise plan with your new dietary choices. It is important to have a clear idea of just what certain types of fuel your body needs for the types of exercise you are interested in continuing but otherwise the most important thing to remember is to eat your biggest meal after you have finished exercising. If your current plan doesn't seem to mix well, that is no reason to lose hope, remember intermittent fasting is all about flexibility, work to find the solution that works best for you.

I can fast successfully during the week but not the weekend, how can I fix this?

It is important to not fixate on intermittent fasting to the point that it becomes more than a guideline. If you find a mix of 16/8 or 20/4 that works for you during the week and then you allow yourself 2 cheat days then this can be perfectly fine, as long as you don't use those days to wreck all of your otherwise successful hard work. It is all about finding what works for you and keeping it up in the long term. It is important to not think of it in terms of the days that you are not sticking with it but to instead consider how successful you are being each and every week day.

Is there anyone who shouldn't try intermittent fasting?

Even something as relatively mild as a 14/10 split shouldn't be attempted by anyone whose body is still growing. Those who are still maturing need all the vitamins and nutrients they can get in order to achieve their maximum potential and even a mild fast now and then could potential lead to issues later in life. Along those same lines, women who are pregnant should forego intermittent fasting until they are no longer pregnant.

Can fasting make me more prone to illness?
As long as you are following a healthy diet that takes into account the vitamins and minerals you are missing out on during your fasting period, then there is no reason that intermittent fasting should ever negatively affect your health. In fact, some studies indicate that indicate the body is more primed and resistant to disease once it has switched to fasting mode.

Is there a way to tell when a type of fasting is the one for me?
While there is no surefire way to know when a type of fasting is the right one for you, the best indicators are typically how hungry you tend to feel at the end of the fasting period and how much energy you have once the fasting phase has started. What it might come down to is that if you don't feel much of anything one way or another after a month of intermittent fasting them maybe you have your answer.

How much should blood glucose decrease in a single week?
Once you are through the transition phase and your body begins to stabilize under its new schedule, it is completely normal for your blood glucose level to decrease by up to 10 mg/dl in a 7-day period. What's more, your blood sugar is also likely to rise each day during the period of time you are fasting before returning to a more normal level after your first meal. This is simply a result of your body

normalizing throughout the day and is nothing to be concerned with.

Conclusion

Thank you again for downloading this book! I hope it was able to help you understand the wide variety of options you have when it comes to intermittent fasting and how you can best mix and match to find the perfect solution for you. Making the decision to alter your primary eating patterns is a major one and it is important that you take the full weight of the decision into account before acting.

With that being said, if you are convinced that you have what it takes to take full advantage of the benefits that intermittent fasting has to offer, then the next step is to stop reading already and to start fasting. Pick the type of intermittent fasting that seems like the best fit for you and give it a try. Don't be discouraged if it doesn't work right away, make an effort to find the one that's right for you. Above all, don't rush; remember, intermittent fasting is a marathon not a sprint, slow and steady wins the race.

Finally, if you enjoyed this book, then I'd like to ask you for a favor, would you be kind enough to leave a review for this book on Amazon? It'd be greatly appreciated!

www.ingramcontent.com/pod-product-compliance
Lightning Source LLC
Chambersburg PA
CBHW061944280526
45787CB00004B/1715